THE HEART AND LUNGS

BODYWORKS

Tracy Maurer

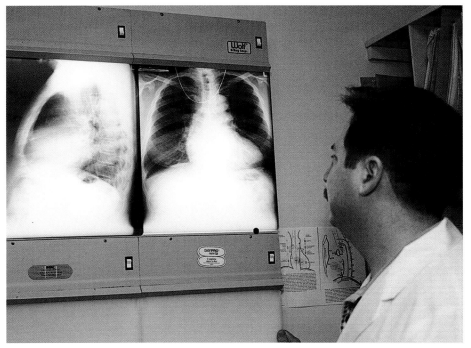

The Rourke Corporation, Inc.
Vero Beach, Florida 32964

Tracy M. Maurer specializes in non-fiction and business writing. Her most recently published children's books include the Let's Dance Series, also from Rourke Pub ishing.

With appreciation to Lois M. Nelson, Dr. Doris Moody - Georgia College and State University, Oconee Regional Medical Center, Mac and Lynn Mitchell, Paige Henson, Drew and Tracy McCroen, and Earl J. Berman, M.D.

PHOTO CREDITS:
All photos © Timothy L. Vacula: except © Lois M. Nelson: page 17

ILLUSTRATIONS: © Todd Tennyson: pages 4, 8

EDITORIAL SERVICES: Janice L. Smith for Penworthy Learning Systems

CREATIVE SERVICES: East Coast Studios, Merritt Island, Florida

Library of Congress Cataloging-in-Publication Data

Maurer, Tracy, 1965-
   The heart and lungs / by Tracy Maurer.
      p. cm. — (Bodyworks)
   Summary: Describes the heart and lungs and how they work together with other parts of the body to help it obtain and use the oxygen it needs.
   ISBN 0-86593-581-5
   1. Cardiopulmonary system Juvenile literature. [1. Respiratory system. 2. Circulatory system.] I. Title. II. Series: Maurer, Tracy, 1965- Bodyworks.
QP103.M28 1999
612.1—dc21   99-23389
                                                                            CIP

Printed in the USA

451 5051

TABLE OF CONTENTS

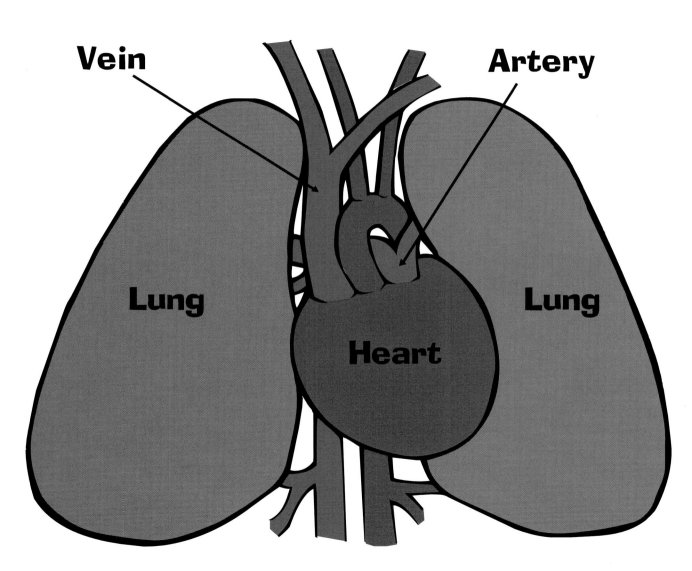

Vein

Artery

Lung

Lung

Heart

THE BODY'S PUMPS

Put your hand on the left side of your chest. Feel your heartbeat. Bah-bump! Bah-bump! Your chest moves up as you breathe in. It moves down as you breathe out.

Humans need the **oxygen** (AHK suh jen) in air to live. The lungs and heart work together to pump oxygen into the blood. Blood carries the oxygen everywhere in the body. Blood also takes the used air, called **carbon dioxide** (KAR ben die AHK side), back to the lungs. There it gets blown out. This is how the **cardiovascular system** (KAR dee oh VAS kyoo ler SIS tim) works.

The heart and lungs form most of the cardiovascular system.

THE AIRWAYS

The nose and mouth connect to an airway in the throat. This airway is called the **trachea** (TRAY key ah). The trachea splits into two main trunks that look like upside-down trees. Each trunk has smaller and smaller branches of airways. They spread across either the left or the right lung.

Muscles around the airways help move the air. Sticky **mucus** (MYOO kus) in the airways traps dust and other harmful specks. Coughing or sneezing helps get rid of the dirty mucus.

The nose and mouth bring oxygen into the body.

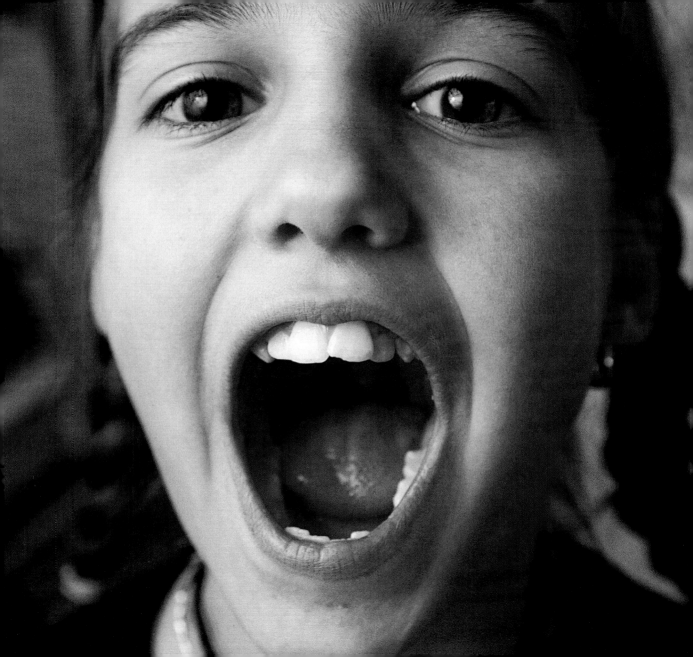

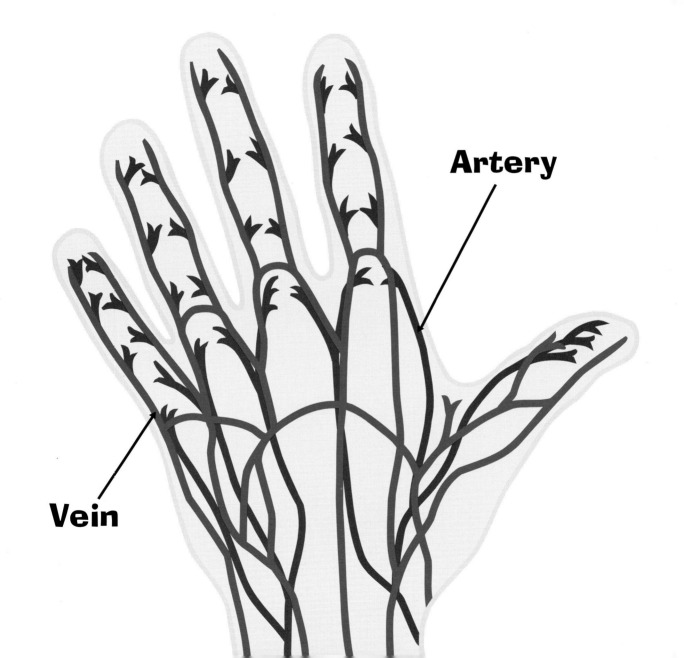

Artery

Vein

ARTERIES AND VEINS

Arteries (AR ter eez) and **veins** (VAYNZ) are the highways for blood. End to end, these tubes would stretch 60,000 miles (96,000 kilometers)! Arteries carry blood away from the heart. Oxygen in the blood colors it bright red. Veins bring the used blood back to the heart. The blood looks blue without oxygen in it.

The heart is a muscle. Although it is not much bigger than a fist, it is very strong. It pumps five quarts of blood in one minute.

Look at the arteries and veins in the drawing. Put your hand over it. Can you see the blue veins in your hand?

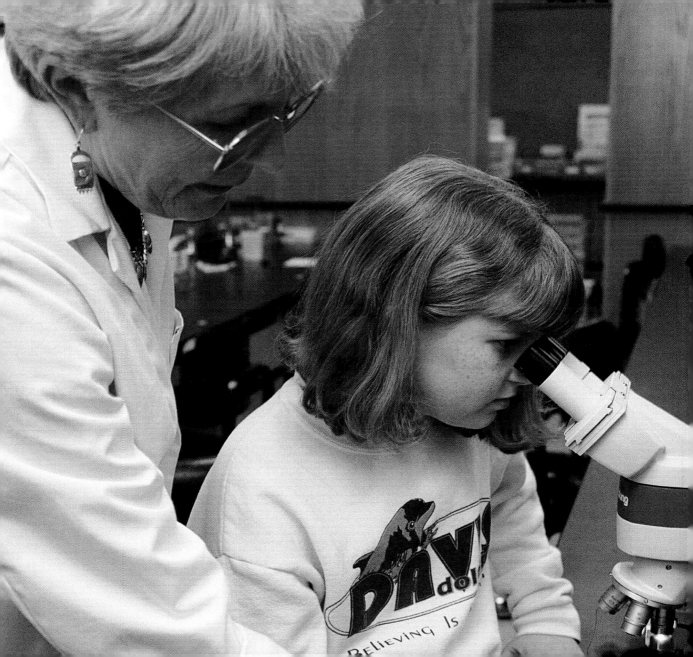

THE BLOOD'S CELLS

The blood contains red and white cells. They do different jobs. Red blood cells pick up oxygen from the lungs. To drop off the oxygen, these cells take turns squeezing through tubes called **capillaries** (KAP ill air eez). The capillaries also pack carbon dioxide into the red cells to take back to the lungs.

White blood cells attack bacteria, viruses and other invaders. Far fewer in number than red blood cells, white blood cells keep us healthy.

This scientist uses a microscope to see red and white blood cells.

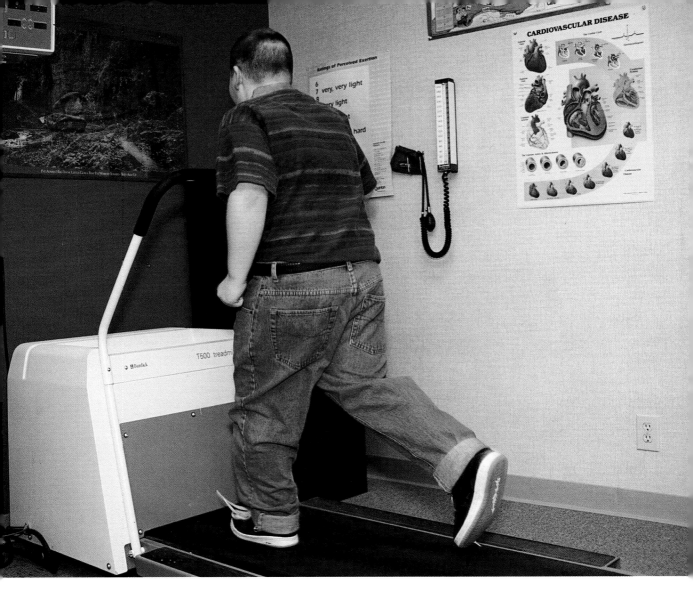

Running on a treadmill makes the heart pump faster. After a patient runs, the doctor listens to the heart and lungs.

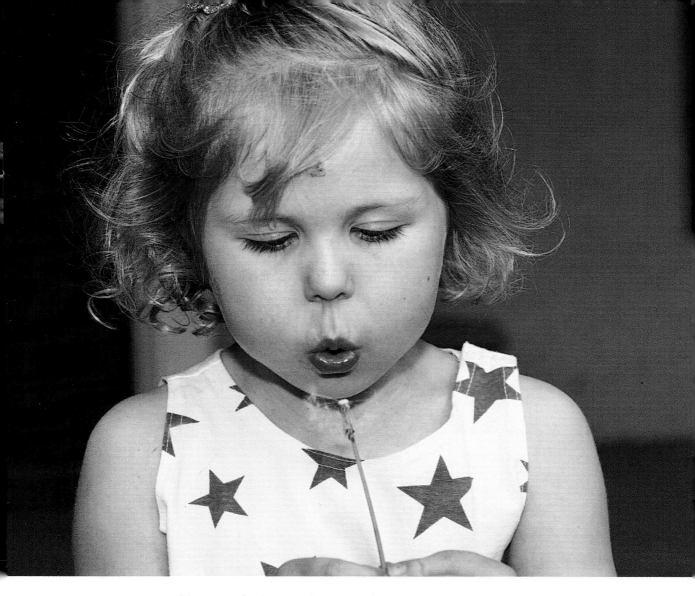

You can feel your chest go down as you blow out air.

WORKING ON THEIR OWN

Your lungs took their first breath when you were born. Your heart started beating even before then! You don't need to think about these functions. Your heart and lungs work without your control.

Special cells inside your heart send out an electrical signal that tells your heart muscle to contract. The muscle relaxes again after the signal passes by. This is a heartbeat. A heart will beat more than two billion times nonstop in a typical lifetime.

A newborn's heart and lungs pump on their own.

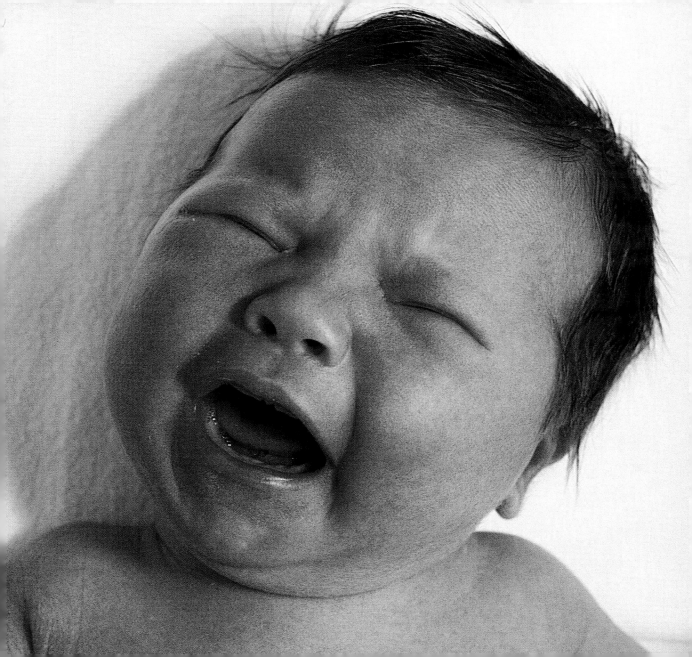

KEEPING UP WITH YOU

Your heart and lungs work all the time. Sometimes they pump faster or slower than usual.

When you run, your muscles want oxygen. Your lungs draw in more air while your heart pumps the blood faster. You breathe harder and your heart beats more quickly!

If you feel cold, your heart and lungs slow down. They may speed up if something frightens you. The heart and lungs meet your needs, even when you sleep.

Your cardiovascular system works harder and faster when you exercise.

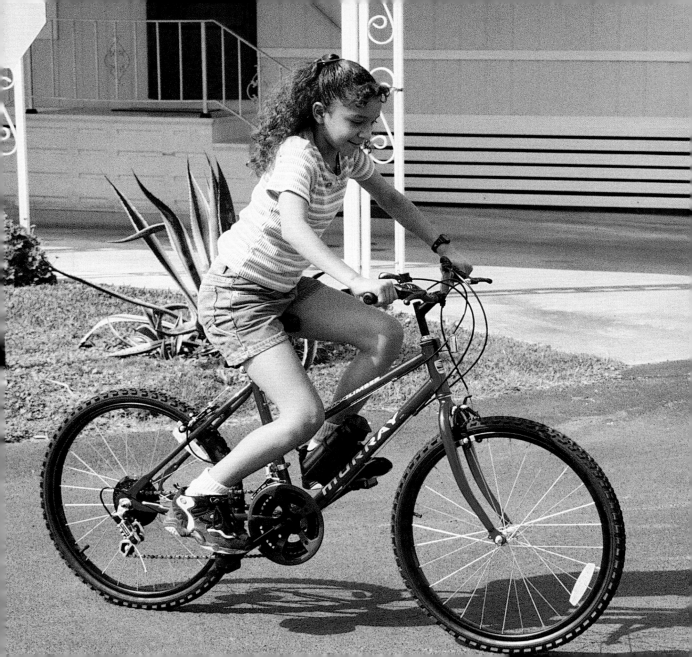

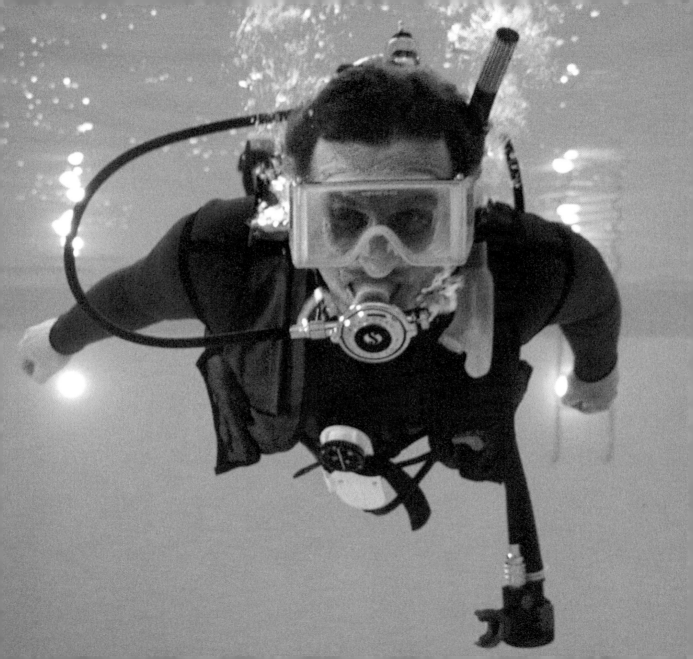

UNDER WATER OR SKY HIGH

Did you know *where* you go can affect your heart and lungs?

A diver's heart may beat more slowly in deeper water. This saves heat and oxygen.

The air in the mountains has less oxygen than air over the sea. In the mountains the heart and lungs must work much harder to take in oxygen at first. After a few days, the body builds up extra red blood cells to carry more oxygen faster.

Deep water feels very cold. A diver's heart and lungs slow down to help keep him warm.

19

ASTHMA ATTACK!

Sometimes the body makes mistakes about its conditions. Children or adults with **asthma** (AZ mah) have sensitive airways. Dust, hot or cold air, exercising, even laughing or crying may cause breathing problems.

During an asthma attack, the muscles tighten around the airways. Extra mucus blocks some of the air. Most people can easily control asthma by breathing in medicine to relax the airway muscles.

Many children have this common lung disease. Fortunately, about half will outgrow it.

About 13 million Americans have asthma. This lung disease can be treated with the right medicine.

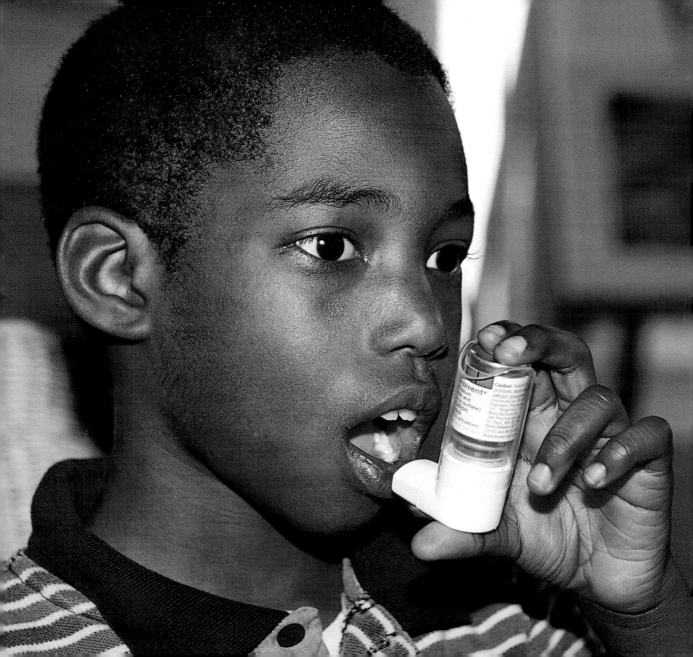

EXERCISE AND EAT RIGHT

The cardiovascular system works better with regular exercise. **Aerobic** (air OH bik) exercise, such as jogging or jumping rope, helps the heart and lungs. It gives these two organs extra practice pumping oxygen into the muscles.

The right foods can also protect your heart and lungs. Too much candy, cookies and cake can lead to blocked arteries. Eat plenty of fruit and vegetables to keep your body healthy. You get only one body. Take good care of it!

GLOSSARY

aerobic (air OH bik) — exercise that makes the heart and lungs work harder to pump blood and oxygen to the body

arteries (AR ter eez) — tubes that carry oxygen-rich blood from the heart to other parts of the body

asthma (AZ mah) — a lung disease causing people to have trouble breathing

capillaries (KAP ill air eez) — tiny tubes that exchange oxygen and carbon dioxide between the arteries and the veins

carbon dioxide (KAR ben die AHK side) — the waste gas people and animals breathe out of their lungs after breathing in oxygen

cardiovascular system (KAR dee oh VAS kyoo ler SIS tim) — the heart, lungs, arteries and veins working together to supply the body with oxygen-rich blood

mucus (MYOO kus) — the body's natural, thick slime

oxygen (AHK suh jen) — a big part of the air people and animals need to breathe in

trachea (TRAY key ah) — the airway from the back of the mouth, down the throat, and into the lungs

veins (VAYNZ) — the tubes that bring blood without oxygen back to the heart

23

INDEX

FURTHER READING:

Find out more about Bodyworks with these helpful books and information sites:

- Walker, Richard. *The Children's Atlas of the Human Body.* Brookfield, Connecticut: The Millbrook Press, 1994.
- Miller, Jonathan, and David Pelham. *The Human Body: The Classic Three-Dimensional Book.* New York: Penguin Books, 1983.
- Williams, Dr. Frances. *Inside Guides: Human Body.* New York: DK Publishing, 1997.

On The World Wide Web
- www.amhrt.org. © American Heart Association, 1997.
- www.lungusa.org. © American Lung Association, 1997.

On CD-ROM
- *The Family Doctor,* 3rd Edition. Edited by Allan H. Bruckheim, M.D. © Creative Multimedia, 1993-1994.